Broken Wings
What's Wrong With Her?

Broken Wings
What's Wrong With Her?

By Stephanie Fortune

Brandylane Publishers, Inc.

ISBN 978-1-883911-93-5

Library of Congress Control Number: 2009944154

Brandylane Publishers, Inc.
www.brandylanepublishers.com

To the memory of my daughter,
Christina Elaine Fortune

Introduction

Christina was born with cerebral palsy and seizures, a disability resulting from lack of oxygen to her brain at birth. This left her unable to walk or talk, and required that she be taken care of twenty-four hours a day. My husband and I were told that she was going to live no more than twenty-four hours after her birth, but as a result of what we believe to be a miracle, this wonderful and loving person lived to be twenty-four years old. She was not only a beautiful young lady; she also carried with her a loving, caring and humble spirit. She spoke no words, but to look at her eyes and see her smile, you knew she was a special child with a sweet soul. Christina enjoyed life as much as her health would allow, and her beautiful spirit touched the lives of many adults and children before and after her death. Of all the questions other children would ask, most of them would ask, "What's wrong with her?"

This is how *Broken Wings* was born.

Broken Wings
What is wrong with her?

I have had many children come to me and take notice of my daughter, Christina. No matter where we were—special occasions, at the mall, in the grocery store, or out to eat. Children who approached me asked all sorts of questions; they would ask why she was in a wheelchair or why is she unable to talk? You know, children have all kinds of questions and they asked them without any hesitation. I always started out telling them that Christina was an angel sent down from Heaven.

It all started one day while we were in the mall. A little girl came to me and asked what happened to Christina. To tell you the truth, I honestly didn't know where this story came from but I just started telling the story to this little girl. I have told this story to many people, and everyone who has listened has reacted with surprise. People have told me that I should write this story down and that it should become a book. As a result of this book, adults and children can, and will, understand Christina's disability.

This is how I have told the story.

Christina was an angel in Heaven. She used to look down at the children on earth and wanted to become a child so desperately. She went to Jesus one day and asked, "Jesus, can I become a little girl today?"

Jesus said, "Precious, no you cannot."

Christina asked, "Jesus, if I cannot become a little girl, then can I become a little boy today?"

He replied, "Oh no, Precious, you cannot become a little boy."

Christina thought and wondered why Jesus was saying no to her questions, so she asked, "Jesus, why can't I become a little boy or girl?"

Jesus replied, "Precious, you are an angel, you are a heavenly angel. You're not a little girl and you're not a little boy."

Christina said, "Well, Jesus I want to become a child on earth so badly, I don't understand why not."

He said, "Precious, you would have to give up a lot to become a child on Earth." Then Jesus asked Christina if she was willing to give up certain advantages to become a child.

"What would I have to give up?" she asked.

He said, "Christina, you would have to give up your wings."

"My wings? My wings are my way of getting around; my wings are my strength," she cried.

Jesus said, "In order for you to become a child, you would have to lose your wings. Look down on Earth. Do you see any of the children with wings?"

Christina looked and said, "No, Father, I don't."

Jesus said, "Children don't have wings. You would have to give up your wings, and giving up your wings, you will lose your ability to fly. You see, the children on Earth do not fly; they walk. You cannot walk because angels fly. If I take your wings away from you, you will not be able to fly or walk."

"Oh Jesus, yes my wings are my strength and without my wings, I cannot do anything," Christina said.

Jesus asked, "Are you willing to give up your wings?" She took her wings and wrapped them around her; she felt the softness and smelled the heavenly scent her wings gave off, and she said, "Oh, good-bye wings; I have to give you up because I want to be a child. With all that is in me, I do, I want to become a child on Earth."

So Jesus said, "If that is what you want, my Precious, that is what you shall have."

Therefore, she stood tall and she turned her back towards Jesus and said, "Father, take them, take my wings, take them right now before I change my mind." She dropped her head and looked down at the children on Earth. She said to herself, *Oh, I do, I do want to become a child*, and Jesus broke off her wings. She fell down on the cloud, weak from losing her wings. She looked up at him and said, "Father, I have no strength. I cannot get up. Is this what my life is going to be like on Earth?" and He said, "Yes, Precious, for you will be a special child. You will be a child who will not be able to walk or hold a spoon to feed yourself and you will be a child who has to eat special food."

She said, "Special food, why?"

"Remember, you are an angel and angels are used to eating angel dust. Therefore, you will not be able to eat solid foods nor chew your food the way children do on Earth," He said. "You will eat, but your food will look a little different from what other people eat. Remember, you are an angel who has given up her wings. You will not have the strength to do anything for yourself. Christina, there is also something else. You will have reactions, reactions that will be called seizures."

"Seizures, Father? I don't understand," she said. Jesus started to explain to her that she was so used to breathing and living in the atmosphere of Heaven that it would be difficult for her to adjust to the way of life and the atmosphere on Earth. In addition, "Another thing, you are going to have to give up your voice," Jesus said. "Give up my voice, Father? But why would I have to do that?" Christina asked. "Because I cannot let you go to Earth and tell what happens here in Heaven. Your mother and father will know and they will let others know that you are special and that you are an angel. Deep inside your heart you know that you are indeed a heavenly angel."

Jesus asked her one last time, "Are you still willing to become a child?" Christina replied, "Father, to give up my wings, to eat special food, to have seizures and to give up my voice, I want to give it all up to become a child on Earth." With this decision, Jesus ran his hand across her mouth and took her voice. With her wings and her voice in his hands, he took both and wrapped a gold string around them, tying them together. Then he put them deep down in his pocket with other beautiful and special good things. He said, "Christina, my number one little one, you may go to Earth as a child now. On Earth you will be a special child, and through your special needs everyone will look at you and will see that you are special. Each person that helps you and shows you kindness will be even closer to Heaven. These people will show you kindness, and you will smile back at them, for you have given up an awful lot. To live as a child you will be an example for others to see."

This is a story I hope will teach children a lesson. When a child sees a person like Christina, he or she will react with compassion. They will say to themselves, "Oh, that's an angel; I need to help that person, let me show that person some kindness." I feel that this is Christina's lesson to each one of us, to show kindness to those who are in need. People and children who are less fortunate than us are truly a gift sent from Heaven. These are special people in so many ways, and we need to be kind and show concern and love. But even more than that, we should also show kindness and love for every person on Earth.

When I told this story to the little girl, her reaction was simply full of compassion. She was so amazed, she said, "Oh my God, an angel! I know an angel and her name is Christina." I walked away lost in the crowd to this little girl and her mother. The mother searched the shopping mall for at least an hour until she found Christina and me in JC Penney. She came to us and said, "Lady, I don't know where you got that story from, but I just wanted to say 'thank you,' because I did not know how to explain to my child the situation of your daughter and so many other people that she sees in wheelchairs. Your story was so good and to the point, you need to write it down. It needs to become a story so that other parents and children, like me, will have a way of explaining to our children the situation of handicapped people."

Heaven – Part 2

Iforgot how good angel's dust tasted. A soft, fluffy, sweet cream made from morning clouds, rain, and sunshine. 'Mmm,' I said to myself as another full spoon of it slid through my lips. As it melted in my mouth, I felt the coolness of the rain. This made me think of Breyer's strawberry ice cream that I truly enjoyed eating. Then there were bits of sunshine that radiated warm waves all through my body. This reminded me of my morning oatmeal. The fluffiness from the clouds took my mind back to the Virginia State Fair, which is where I got my first taste of cotton candy. As angel Glorious—the angel who is taking care of Christina—was about to give me another spoon full of splendor, I heard someone saying, "Not another bite, two bowls are quite enough, don't you think my number one little one? 'Number one little one,' I thought. I have not been called that name in quite sometime. The only one that addresses me as 'number one little one' is Jesus. "Don't give her another spoonful," He said to Glorious, "Christina, welcome back." He sat down along side my bed, made of clouds, and took my hand. "The Heavens missed you, I missed you." The choir has not sounded the same without you, its tiny bell ringer. The meadows don't seem as bright, they miss your individual care," Jesus said. It was wonderful to see Jesus. I heard everything he was saying but I was thinking about my parents and what was happening with them.

"I know your thoughts, Christina," Jesus said, "and understand what's going on in your head. Your heart is so overwhelmed with your feelings, but they will soon turn into joy. Your family has to bear the pain and the distress of your death. They will grieve for a long time in deep sorrow, for they will miss you very much. Christina, your time on Earth is finished and it is time to reclaim your heavenly body. Little one, your eyes say so much, and soon you will be able to tell your story." Jesus picked me up from my cloud and held me close to him. He said to me, "I know your most inner feelings and the need for you to say good-bye. The disconnection from earthly living is not easy to let go of when there is so much love keeping it connected."

I closed my eyes and just felt the comfort of being in his arms. Lying in his comfort, my mind became at ease and I began thinking about my life. My thoughts reminded me of having cerebral palsy and of my seizures. These two illnesses may have entangled my body, but my mind and heart took in all of what my parents allowed my life to be. These things I did not want to forget. Life was good; my parents were wonderful. I had the joy of family and friends. I met many good people and bad, I was shown lots of places; some places I enjoyed and some I did not. I ate delicious tasting food and some not so tasty. I enjoyed music of all kinds. I enjoyed fun moments and others that were not. My parents did not let life abandon me. There were times that I will forget. While I was sick, there were too many hard days and nights. My mother's loving, caring ways allowed me to recover from my illnesses with the strength to go on.

At that moment, Jesus asked me to open my eyes. We were back in my hospital room. I then remembered feeling sick and going into a seizure. I remembered the doctors and the nurses. There were many things happening to me and around me. There was so much confusion, so much discomfort. There was my father kissing me and rubbing my head, my grandmother holding my hand and telling me she loved me. I could see my uncle Rodney; he was so upset. I wanted to tell him, "I'm going to be all right, Uncle Rodney. Please don't cry." The medication they are giving me is making me feel better. There was my Aunt Gail. She always made me smile. Just to think of her made me have involuntary explosive sounds of laughter. I wish we could get some laughter in this room and do away with all this sadness.

"You are right with that thought," Jesus said, "but there will not be any laughter here. Reflect on the serious mind-set of your family. They know they are standing in the moment of death. Look at your mother, and listen to what she is saying to you." At that moment there was a pain in my heart. My chest felt like something heavy was sitting on me. This was a pain like nothing I had experienced before. My body was so weak it could not respond to the pain. I then realized I was back in my body and being pulled by my mother to her chest. I heard her say as she kissed my forehead, "It's okay, Sugar, let go. Mama's going to be all right. The angels are here to take you back to Heaven. Remember Mama, Sugar, I love you."

With my last struggle before death, I tried to give her love. With that said, I looked and there were angels in my room. As my mother laid me down, the angels came closer to my bed and I saw Jesus sitting with his arms reaching out to me. One angel lifted my spirit from my body and placed me in the arms of Jesus.

"Suffer the little children for they shall come unto me," Jesus spoke. He looked down at me and smiled. He said once again, "Suffer little children for they shall come unto me." As he touched me from the very top of my head to the tips of each of my fingers and to the very tip of each toe, I felt the strength entering me. He kissed my lips and I said clearly, "Thank you." He brought me to my feet; there was a feeling that was long since gone; the feeling of strength and the ability, once again, to feel vigorous and strong. I had to stop and take notice of my family; their sadness overtook me. "What can I do?" I said to Jesus. "This is their moment to observe death," He said.

"I want to go to them," I said. "Then you need to have these," He said. Then he gave me back my wings. They still had the most delightful smell, the most pleasant odor that Heaven only embellished. I marvel over my wings; they were brilliant white, soft and gorgeous. Then the angels surrounded me and with the blink of an eye there I stood all anew, dressed in a long loose, flowing white garment. I felt and was very spiritual. I took the hands of Jesus and said a prayer of thanksgiving. "Go to them," He said. I flew over to my parents. They were still looking over my lifeless body, both of them holding back their tears. I was in midair over them. I put my left hand on my mother's right shoulder. I placed my right hand on my father's left shoulder. With what energy I had, I enforced my love and thanks to both of them. I kissed both of them on their head and said, "I love you both."

"It's time, little one, to leave here," Jesus said. I flew over and stood along side Him with the other angels. Jesus put his left arm around my shoulders, turned me around, and said, "You are not to look back. Your body is dead. It will be buried and in time forgotten. In the hearts of your parents you will live. Your parents, family, and friends that know and love the Lord will come into death and their souls will live with you in Heaven. For now the life of Christina Elaine Fortune, born June 27, 1979 to William and Stephanie Fortune, is finished."

The room felt as if thunder shook it. As I stood with my life behind me, the hospital wall disappeared, vanished before me. There was the open sky; it was the color of the bluest ocean, the sun so luminous with its warm cheerful rays. There were white clouds floating above.

Jesus took me by my hand and we walked out from my hospital room onto a pathway that was green with lush grass. The smell of fresh morning dew was all around me. I looked and there were other souls coming along with us. Angels were holding infants and angels holding the hands of young children. Once again, I heard and felt the sound of thunder. It was Jesus saying, "Forbid them not the Kingdom of Heaven." As we walked, I could hear the sound of angels singing. I looked around we were surrounded by nothing but beauty, so pleasing to the eye. There I stood in a meadow with clear running streams; an aurora beam of light shooting up from the horizon and a steady flow of fresh sweet air. There were beautiful animals of all shapes and sizes. There were beautiful flowers and trees. The birds sing with heart-filled songs. They sang as if in tune with the songs of the angels. As I stood there once again trying to take it all in, I saw my great-grandma Julia standing in front of me with open arms. I thought to myself as she embraced me, she still had that wonderful smell of chocolate cake. Along with her were my grandparents, William and Mable Fortune. "You grew up to be a lovely young lady," they said. I got hugs and kisses from each of them. As we walked along talking of past events and of the wonders of this special place, we came up on my cousin Cameron and my Grandpa Joe. From them I got more hugs and kisses. I saw more family, friends, and classmates from long ago. Running and jumping for butterflies were my dogs Piccalo, Cece, and Buttons. There were people all around that were full of beauty, peace, and happiness. It all suddenly came clear to me; this was my beginning, the place that I call "Heaven."

Close Friends Express Their Thoughts
with Loving Words of Christina

My Special Child

The smile in my child's eyes definitely says it all. She need not learn to speak, we communicate with our hearts and minds. She knows how much I love her; she knows how much I care. She taught me this for I was new to love so deep. It is surreal to the depth of my soul. I love to make her laugh with my goofy grin as she watches me from her chair. For my child is a gift from God, this I know. I knew she was not like other children; she was born with special needs. I knew she would never run and play like other kids. I knew she would not grow up and be the first woman president. No, I did not resent other parents or their precious children who were normal. I know now that God gives special babies to special parents like me.

Thank you for choosing me, my child, Christina, my angel.

Love, Patty
a family friend

To Christina

You hold tight clutched
In cool unknowing little palms
A seed of all innocence;
Eyes straining alertness, response,
Deep brown irises
Mutely mirror dark suns
Your tiny frame
A sweet wasteland of passion—
So small, so weakly miniscule
You bend your back
(Strong with unmerited suffering)
Beneath Simon's wood
(Alike un-volunteered)
Therefore, our sinful world
Is again subtly redeemed

From Paul, a family friend

Christina

The breath she needed to take at birth to begin her life she could not take on her own, but she took them as her last breath before her life ended. The birth cord around her neck at birth constricted her airway and she had to be put in an incubator. Her last moments before death, I held her in my arms and she took three breaths and then passed over into the arms of Jesus. She put forth great efforts throughout her life to live. She struggled with seizures, pneumonia, and by having cerebral palsy, her struggle became a battle she was not going to lose. She fought everyday of her life. Christina was strong and a fighter; most of all, she was indeed a child of God and she was not about to let Satan in any way have a moment of control over her. I thank God for her. I knew she would be blessed with a mission. I believe her mission was to save lives, which included her father and I and all who came into her life. I truly believe that when she stood before our Lord, she had a list of names to give Him. Christina was her chosen name, but Angelic also suited her. It was used twice to describe her: in the beginning of her life and at the end. Angelic female is what was written in her birth report. After her death, the doctor stated how angelic she was, and once again, it was written "Angelic female." When the nurse entered her room, she stopped and said, "My God, the Angels are taking her now." Angelic and blessed by God with eternal innocence is how I feel. I am so thankful that others saw in her the spiritual personality she had.

Her body was not placed in the morgue on the night of her passing. The doctor wrote the order to wash and dress Christina in her nightgown and to let her stay in the bed until morning when the funeral home came to retrieve her body. "Angels are in this room," the doctor said, "I will not disturb this peace. She is not to be placed in the morgue." My mother went back to her room before leaving the hospital to visit with her once more. She said that if you were just passing by her room and looked in, you would have thought she was simply sleeping. Angels were there in the nurses unit that night. The whole wing was very still, and everyone noticed a spirit of peace on the floor. It was not easy for me to walk away from her that night. The Holy Spirit spoke to me and said, "It's over, go home." I felt His hand on my back, pushing me to the door. I felt Christina's soul leave her body, then I knew she was gone. What else was there for me to do but walk away?

The next day was Monday morning. My husband and I had to be at the funeral home by noon. I was sick to my stomach with intestinal distress. I asked God if He would please help me. "How am I going to be able to bury my child," I asked. "God, please give me the strength," I said as I sat down at my kitchen table placing my head in my hands. The Spirit began to speak to me saying, "You are to go to the funeral home and you are to make sure everything is just the way you want it. Christina's body is dead. You are to remember that her spirit is with me. You are to bury her body and let her go." At that moment, I got a feeling in my body that I cannot explain. I got a pen and paper together and started writing out her obituary. "Short and sweet," I said to my husband. "I want everything short and sweet." I got her clothes and make-up together. My husband and I made the arrangements. Christina and her funeral were so beautiful. It was hard to believe that so much beauty came out of a week of storms. Christina died on Sunday, and early Monday morning, a tornado hit the north side of the city. We had also been hit with a hurricane on the Wednesday before her death. Richmond had devastation all around, but God had His hand in everything. Her funeral was at 12:00 noon on September 23rd, and it was a most beautiful day. The air was warm and fresh and the sun was a bright yellow gold, not a cloud in the sky. The birds filled the air singing their songs; butterflies and bees were all around. It was like a spring morning. Surely, gifts from God, "a special day for a special girl," people said. I am so thankful for God and the presents He put in my life and for blessing me with my special child.

When my husband and I had been told that Christina had suffered brain damage at birth, we were both devastated. She was our first and only child. Had I done something wrong? I ate all the right things: vegetables, fruits, drank plenty of milk, water and juices. I took those bad tasting pre-natal vitamins everyday. We were told the umbilical cord had somehow wrapped itself around her neck. As she was being born, the umbilical cord drew tighter and collapsed her airway, and she suffered physical and mental strain that lead to her cerebral palsy. Moments after her birth, she started having seizures which came from the lack of oxygen to the brain. She had been without oxygen for more than four minutes. She was placed on a respirator for a few days until she was able to breath on her own. The doctor started her on seizure medication which she took three times a day for the rest of her life. She started first on a medication called Phenobarbital and Tegretol. In later years, her medication changed numerous times. She took Celontin, Neurontin, Trileptal, Topamax and Keppra, just to name a few. I called Neurontin her miracle drug. For a while, Dr. Pellock was having trouble controlling her seizures. At the time, he wanted to try a new drug, hoping it would get her seizures under control, and it did; she would go for weeks without a seizure. She would be on Neurontin for the rest of her life.

She suffered severe seizures during her teenage years as well. It was because her body was changing. She was going through puberty. When she started her periods or the medical term, pre-menstrual cycles, I believe we both went through pain. Christina's pain was in her stomach and mine was in my heart. She was growing up and her body was no longer a little girl's. Her body frame remained small and I truly thank God for that. I talked to Christina previously about little girls becoming young women. I do believe she understood me, but when it finally happened, she was in pain. I was in disbelief and a great loss. I called Dr. Battista, my gynecologist, and he saw Christina right away. He started giving her a new medication called Depo-Provera. This shot—a form of birth control that stopped her menstrual cycle—was given to her every three months. Fortunately, this new drug had no serious side effects, which was my biggest concern. Christina did exceptionally well with this treatment. After her doctors' visits, we always ended with a treat. She looked forward to this each time. After giving the shot, her nurse would say, "Christina, are you going for your strawberry milkshake?" Christina would kick out her right leg, push her body back, and then give the nurse a chuckle. One thing about Christina, she did not fret about receiving her shots or medications. She understood it all was for her well-being. In her special way of chuckling, I believe she was saying, "Bring it on." The treat was my way of saying I was sorry she had to go through so much pain. I would sit still, hold her in my arms like a baby and rock her back and forth.

I remember while rocking her that devastating office visit to see Dr. Pellock. I knew something was wrong when Christina was five months old and was unable to hold her head up or roll over from side to side. I was not ready to hear what the doctor was about to tell me. "Retarded" is what he said. I could not bear to hear that word and it still hurts when I hear it today. I would never allow that word to be used in my presence or Christina's describing her mental development. Mental delay is how I would say it. I asked all of her teachers and therapists never to use the word retarded to describe my daughter, and nobody ever did, not even her doctors.

Christina began special education school at the age of six months. She stayed in special education until she turned twenty-two years old. At that time, she graduated from King William High School. Her first school was Hickory Hills, where a new program was being offered for children with special needs. It was a wonderful program and very helpful to Christina. There, she was around other children like herself. They all received physical therapy, occupational therapy, swimming, speech therapy, all with one-on-one care. It took Christina years to improve her fine motor skills. One thing about Christina was that she was very determined to work hard. While at Hickory Hills, Christina became the schools spokeschild. It was true, she could not speak a word, but she spoke with her presence. She was asked to represent her school on a talk show called FYI (For Your Information). My child was a TV star at the early age of eight months old. Christina and her teachers got the word out on national TV about the need for special education. Her father and I were indeed proud parents that day and everyday of her life.

Christina did not like being still; she liked going outdoors, especially early mornings and late evenings. When the weather was good, we would sit outside in the morning to wait for the school bus. She was always excited about school. She enjoyed going to school when she was able to go. If the weather was nice, we went for a stroll after dinner. There was just something about strolling among the trees that she loved. She would look up at a tree with a look of WOW! and would get so excited when we strolled over dry leaves when they made that crunching sound. After her death, I got a letter from the National Forest Association saying they had planted a tree in her honor for The Living Memorial Program. I am happy to know that someone other than me knew she loved nature. I am also thankful to that person for such a wonderful thing they did to honor Christina.

Christina was my joy, my life, my child. She loved to eat good tasting food. She seemed to savor the flavors with every small spoonful. I fed her with a rubber spoon. I would never ever feed her with plastic. I had a fear that she would bite the plastic and become badly injured from broken plastic in her mouth and stomach. Her nourishment was important to me because I believed in good health for her; she received her medication through her food and juices.

Christina also loved beautiful things, TV and music. She loved small handbeaded handbags, silks and perfumes, along with lipstick. Going to the mall was for Friday nights and weekends. *CNN News* and *Judge Joe Brown* is what she liked to watch on TV. As for music, she liked jazz and Yanni. The groundskeeper at her school played *Amazing Grace* on his saxophone during her funeral. He knew that jazz was her favorite music and he blew that sax from the heart just for her, he said. It was beautiful and makes my heart feel so good to think back on how people loved my daughter.

Christina was a small dainty young lady of forty-eight pounds, 4 feet and 5½ inches tall. She had to have complete care and was wheelchair bound. She was, in a nutshell, sweetness. Everyone noticed that sweetness wherever she went. We were out one Friday night with family planning a trip to Disneyland for Christina's 18th birthday. A very nice woman at the table beside ours had overheard our plans. When she finished her dinner, she came over to our table, gave Christina a small sum of money, and said this is for your birthday trip and I pray that you will have a wonderful time. Later that year, we saw her again at dinner and she was happy to hear that Christina indeed had a wonderful birthday trip to Disneyland.

Christina's way of communicating was through her eyes, kicking her legs and making her coo sounds. Christina was sensitive to emotions; if she noticed your negative feelings, right in your presence, she would simply close her eyes and would keep them closed until you were no longer around. If you were a pleasant person, she loved being in your company. Her excitement was heard in her coo sounds. If her coo was high pitched and one after another, this was excitement. If she made the sound somewhat of a low coo that seemed like a cry, this meant something was wrong; she was not content with herself or with her surroundings or just simply wet and uncomfortable and needed a change. I would say to her, "What's wrong with Mama's Sugar?" I would then give her a kiss under her chin, remove her from the wheelchair and take care of her problem. All she would look for was love and care. Her father and I made sure she got it.

For a little girl, you would think pink, lavender, and blue or maybe yellow could be one of her favorite colors. Oh no, not Christina! Her favorite color was lime green. I found that out one Saturday morning when she and I were out shopping for an Easter outfit for her to wear. We came across a two-piece suit in Sears. I happened to pull it from the rack just to see what it was. It was so loud and flat out ugly, but to my little girl, she started to kick her legs vigorously. Her coo was loud and strong. Her facial expression was full of happiness. It was clear that the ugly florescent lime green suit with white butterflies was the outfit of her choice. She just about came up out of her wheelchair when I said, "I don't think so, Christina," putting it back on the rack. "It's not about you, is it?" I heard someone say. A woman had come over to her and said, "With all this excitement, I see you like lime green." Christina had that look of pleasure in her face as the woman placed the outfit up to her. "Are you going to buy it for her or shall I?" she asked. "Please allow me to do this for her. I enjoyed so much seeing her very excited." Before that shopping day was over, Christina had also gotten a pair of white sunglasses, white stockings and a pair of white sandals to match her florescent lime green Easter outfit. When that Easter Sunday morning came, she looked absolutely stunning for Easter.

Christina had a nickname given to her by her Aunt Gail. Pissy Chrissy is what she called her. It is not that she smelled of urine; it was because she wore pampers. "I'm just teasing you," Gail would say, and Christina didn't seem to mine. Christina was the only female granddaughter in the family at the time. The grandchildren were Gail's two boys and Christina. Christina's cousins were Cameron and Jamie. Cameron was about eight, Jamie five or six and Christina, seven years of age. I remember one summer weekend when the boys stayed over. They loved spending time with Christina and would fight over who was going to push her wheelchair. That Saturday afternoon, we were all in the house taking a nap before going to the movies later that evening. I thought they were all asleep so I tried to get a little nap, too. I later got up to check on Christina and they were not in their beds, in the house or outside, and I was frantic wondering what has happened. Where are Christina and the boys? I was on the phone with my sister, Marjorie and was about to call the police when she said to look outdoors and check with the neighbors. I was just about to do that when I looked out the front door and there they were, coming down the street. Cameron was pushing the wheelchair, Jamie was walking alongside holding Christina's hand, and all three were grinning from ear to ear. Christina's mouth was blue from sucking on a straw that contained grape powder Kool-Aid. Jamie's mouth was red with no front teeth that held a large red blow-pop sucker. Cameron's chest was stuck out as if he had done the greatest thing in the world. He had taken his brother and cousin to the store for candy. As I rushed out the door, I suddenly started to laugh. They looked so funny, so happy, and they were safe. After seeing those faces, I could not stay upset with them. Cameron said he asked me if it was all right and I said that it was fine. Now remember, I was asleep at the time. It's no telling what I said. Still, I was proud of him for getting her up from her bed and placing her correctly in the wheelchair. He gave each of them something to drink before they started out to the store. He knew what to do and he did it all just right. How could I stay upset? I'm sorry I did not get a picture of all of this. They were happy and Christina was a sticky mess. She clearly enjoyed every bit of that adventure.

Cameron and Christina looked more like sister and brother. Throughout their lives, both Cameron and Jamie were very attentive to her. Cameron went to live with his father in Boston at an early age, and when he came home for the holidays, he was sure to visit with Christina. Unfortunately, Cameron died accidentally at the age of twenty-five. Christina rests along beside him, and they have matching headstones. For every holiday and for each season, I change their flowers. I stand there with my memories of each of them. Both of them were beautiful people with beautiful souls, and I try to keep their resting place beautiful, too. Jamie was Christina's protector and was always telling her how pretty she was and how he would fight a person if they tried to hurt her. He has two sons of his own. Sadly, their mother was killed in a car accident, also at the age of twenty-five.

Christina had a crush on her high school teacher, Mr. Shipman, a dear and wonderful man. He took good care of not only Christina, but all his students. Every one of the students loved Mr. Shipman. The night of Christina's prom, he made sure everything was just right for her. It truly was a special night. Christina and her date, David, wore black and white, offset by a half dozen yellow roses given to her by David and picked out by Mr. Shipmen. For some reason, he knew she liked yellow roses. He gave me one dozen long stem yellow roses in a crystal vase at Christina's funeral. He called Christina his little chick-a-dee. He was the only one that could get her to eat her lunch at school. Christina had to be fed. She was not able to do it herself. She would not eat for anyone else. He would eat together with Christina everyday. Everyday he would share his Coca Cola with her, and then she would eat her lunch. If for some reason Mr. Shipman missed school, Christina would not eat her lunch. She looked forward to her one-on-one lunchtime with him. He was her teacher for four years—a remarkable special education teacher and indeed a wonderful man. Mr. Shipman had two students—Christina and another student—to pass away within a year's time, and he also lost a dear friend, Mrs. Ball, the high school principal who was also a friend of mine. These deaths, along with personal problems, took a toll on him and he committed suicide. How sad that nobody saw the pain in him, including myself. I saw him a week before he took his own life. He seemed his usual happy self. Mr. Shipman and I talked about Christina and other things for about an hour then we hugged and said our good-byes. I am sorry I did not know that my friend was in such pain. I'm glad that I did get to talk to him for that short hour. He was a very good teacher and good to my daughter and good to me.

Christina was a fighter and she worked hard to maintain skills that took her years to master. I remember how hard it was for her to eat. One thing she loved the most was food. With spastic arms, it was hard for her to hold a spoon. She was able to have more control as the years passed, but she never was able to feed or care for herself. A therapist told her that she would never be able to suck from a straw. I had asked the question about a straw because I saw other kids using the straw as part of their therapy. "Why couldn't Christina?" I asked. It was because she could not close her mouth around the straw. Sucking from a straw will never be an option for her. "Never be an option for my Christina," I said. "I think not"—and that night, we started working on sucking from a straw. I saw the sadness in her face with the first few tries. "We are not giving up and will work on this every night, okay, Sugar?" Then she would look at me with a pretty little smile. In about two weeks, I came to school with Christina and had her breakfast with us. "We have something to show the teachers and therapist," I said. I made a warm oatmeal strawberry milkshake. I placed a flexible straw in the mug and placed it into Christina's mouth. She started sucking the oatmeal through the straw. "Well done!" said her teacher. "I can't believe she was able to do that," said the therapist who said in the beginning that Christina would never be able to do it. "Show us the technique you used and tell us what's in the mug. It must be good because she drank the whole mug."

I explained that the first thing I do is take a blender and chop up the oatmeal until it becomes fine; then cook the oatmeal in milk, butter and sugar with just a pinch of cinnamon. I pour it into a mug and add pureed strawberries and milk, then place the flexible straw on the middle of her tongue and take my thumb and place it just under her bottom lip and my pointer finger and place it over her top lip to close her mouth around the straw. I would then squeeze her nose closed for just a second so that she would inhale through her mouth to get the flow of the oatmeal through the straw. Again, I stress just a second because I did not want her to aspirate from holding her nose. I did not want the food to go into her lungs. Once she got the taste of food and the feel of the straw, she began to do it herself whenever the straw was placed on her tongue. Everyone was so impressed with her, they recorded it on film to teach other therapists. Christina succeeded in something that she was told would never happen. She liked using the straw for breakfast shakes and smoothies. (*All of Christina's favorite recipes are available in the back of the book*).

Christina liked being in the kitchen and helping me cook. She loved eating, tasting and smelling good food. She liked putting her hands directly into the mix or hamburger and using the hand-held mixer. She liked keeping herself active in the kitchen and in the household chores. Keeping her involved made her feel needed and we all wanted her to feel that she was needed. Washing dishes was the ultimate thing she loved to do. She enjoyed having her sleeves pushed up her arms and her hands in soapy dishwater. I would put a pillow up against the sink for her to rest on and then let her kneel in a chair that I pushed up to the sink sideways so I could stand and support her from behind. I then would place her hands in the water with my hands to support the plate and together we would wash the plates. She would keep a serious look on her face the whole time. After everything was done, she gave me that pretty little smile as if to say, thank you mama for helping me.

She would also give me that special smile after a good hot bath. This too, along with getting her hair washed, was a favorite thing to do. Bath time indeed was very special to her. There was something about hot soapy water. Sometimes she would get into the tub with me. We would lay back and soak in a warm bath filled with bubbles. After soaking for a few minutes, I would then bathe her then my husband would come and take her out of the water to dry her off with a towel. Other times, I would lay towels and chucks over the counter at the sink in the kitchen, then I would lay her down on the towels with her feet resting in the warm soapy water in the sink and give her a bath. After bath time, I would wrap her in a nice clean towel and turn her the other way at the kitchen sink to wash her hair. After I washed her hair, I would take her to the bedroom, place her on a large towel that was on the bed, rub her dry from head to toe, put lotion on her, and sprinkle her with a sweet powder. I would never put fragrances on her personal area. From her scalp to her pretty little toes, I only used Pond's hydrating skin cream or original Keri dry skin lotion to moisturize her skin. Christina's perfume was Youth-Dew by Estee Lauder and for her body cream, I would only use a very small amount whenever I put it on her. The body cream is very strong and you don't want to use too much. Christina loved it and it smelled wonderful on her. After bath time was over, I would put her in her wheelchair and take her to the kitchen to give medication to her and a bowl of warm mashed fruit. The warm mashed fruit helped with constipation. After the small glass of juice, I would let her watch TV and then off to bed about 10:00 pm. Some nights I read to her from books like *Jane Eyre* or *Great Expectations*. These two were the books she liked the most. As I said before, I gave her mashed warm fruit for constipation because Christina suffered with constipation, which could trigger seizures. Every night I gave this to her along with her medication in a bowl of cooked fruit like prunes, strawberries, apricots, peaches and apples cooked in apple juice. These mashed fruits were also added to oatmeal, yogurt and ice cream for milkshakes. Wednesday nights I would have to give her an enema. She never fussed about it and she understood what I told her, that it was helping her stomach to feel better and when her stomach felt better, she felt better. I would warm the enema by placing it in a cup of warm water for a few minutes before giving it to her. I then put a large amount of Vaseline over her rectum, which helped the stool to pass through with ease. Then I would give the enema to her on the bed. After a few minutes, I took her to the bathroom and there, I placed a chair with a pillow on the back of the chair for me to rest my back against. Remember, she could not sit up on her own. This is why I had the chair pushed up against the toilet so I could sit on the chair while holding her over the toilet. I did it both ways, one with her facing the toilet or the other way with her facing me. If she was facing the toilet, she could rest her back against my chest and my arms would be around her for support. Her legs hung over my thighs beside the toilet, which kept her elevated from the cold, hard toilet seat. She did her business while facing me and giving me a big hug. It was more at ease for her in this position because sometimes she would go to sleep.

I am happy to say that Christina never got upset about anything. I would explain everything I could to her so she would understand. She would not get upset about her appointments to the doctor's office, because she understood the reason why she had to see the doctors. She knew that nobody likes being in the hospital but she was brave and endured everything with courage and grace. She knew it was in her best interest at that time to stay healthy. Any tests she had to go through, the doctors and I explained it to her. After everything she had been through, I felt that it was necessary to explain everything to her in detail. She needed to be treated like the person she is—a human being—and not be discarded and put aside just because she had a handicap.

My husband and I did the very best we could do for Christina during her life. We made sure we gave her the best of the world. We were blessed to be given such a special child. In my heart, I feel she was a spiritual being. She was given to me to save my soul, as well as the soul of others. I believe this because in her eyes shined the brightness of the strength of her soul. Her smile showed you that she was blessed with eternal innocence. She was a gift from God and you had to respect that and understand it if you know Him. God has many ways of doing things. This He did for me, by giving me my special child, and I am thankful for being her mother. Christina had a difficult life of being a person that had the need of total care, enduring the illness of seizures. Through this, she still maintained a pleasant spirit. "Suffer the children to come unto me and forbid them not, for of such is the kingdom of God." This is what God said, as written in the Bible. This is where my Christina is today. Heaven!

Angels Have Daily Needs, Too!
Tips On How I Cared for My Special Angel!

Children and adults with special needs cannot always communicate what their needs are or what is uncomfortable, so it is our job to make sure that everything is pain free and comfortable. Here are some suggestions for those caring for special needs children.

Bath: In the morning, I would only give Christina a sponge bath. I would wash her face, underarms, bottom and her back. This was especially important because she slept on her back. After washing her with warm water and Dove soap, I would put lotion on her using Keri or Ponds lotion. Keri lotion is the best and Ponds Moisturizing Cream is excellent for skin care. I would only wash her with Dove soap as it gave her beautiful skin. I used it on her for as long as I can remember. I believe Dove to be best for people who spend long periods sitting or lying down, as it's good for sensitive skin. I used the lotions and creams on her from the top of her head to the tip of her toes.

I gave Christina baths twice a week—on Sundays and on Wednesday night. Her complete bath consisted of washing her hair and submersion of her body in bath water. I would wash her hair with Pantene Shampoo and Conditioner, and to keep her scalp from drying out, I used Ponds Moisture. Due to the headrest on her wheelchair, I did not use barrettes, rubber bands, hairpins or anything on the back or the sides of Christina's head, as these things would keep her from having freedom of head movement and make her uncomfortable. If I put any on her, I would put them on top of her head and even at that, I put them on her very loosely. I did not want anything to cause her to have any headaches. Even when a headrest was being used, I did not put earrings on her, as it would cause some discomfort, as well. The earrings would cause redness, soreness and swelling to the ear lobes and sometimes infection to her ears.

I never used inexpensive diapers on her. It was very important to me to make sure she was comfortable, so I made sure the diapers fit her around the legs and the elastic was not too tight so it would not cut into her legs. I also made sure they were not too tight around her belly. I never used baby wipes on her, only soap and water. When she had a bowel movement, I would only use Keri Lotion or Ponds Cream because this would keep the skin soft and it also easily removed the waste. Christina never had a diaper rash or skin breakage on her bottom.

Deodorant: Christina would have Avon Skin-So-Soft used on her for sensitive skin.

Teeth: She had regular dental check-ups. Christina's teeth were so beautiful. I used a soft toothbrush using Crest toothpaste and very little mouthwash was mixed with a little water. She liked Scope Mint mouthwash. After I brushed her teeth, I mixed a ½ cap full of mouthwash with a little water in a cup. Then I rinsed the toothbrush, dipped it into the mouthwash and started all over again to brush her teeth a second time using the mouthwash; then I gave her a little cup of cool water to drink.

Powder: I never put powder on her bottom or her Pampers. I only put powder on her chest and stomach areas. She loved the smell of Esteé Lauder's Youth Dew.

Bra: I did not put a bra on Christina. She would only wear a camisole or a body-shape top under her clothes. If she needed to wear a bra, I would use one with no underwire, no metal on the straps, and with front closure only. The metal would have a tendency to cut into her skin (we all want to be comfortable).

Clothing: The only fabrics I put on Christiana were cotton, jersey, knit, fleece, micro-fleece and soft pre-washed denim. I liked her to wear soft light color clothing at all times. In the summer, she wore a lot of seersucker with a light cotton fabric. Light colors gave her a clean crisp look and would keep her cool

Christina's class at Virginia Randolph Special Education Center, Richmond, Virginia created this book in honor of Christina. We are recreating it here in remembrance of her.

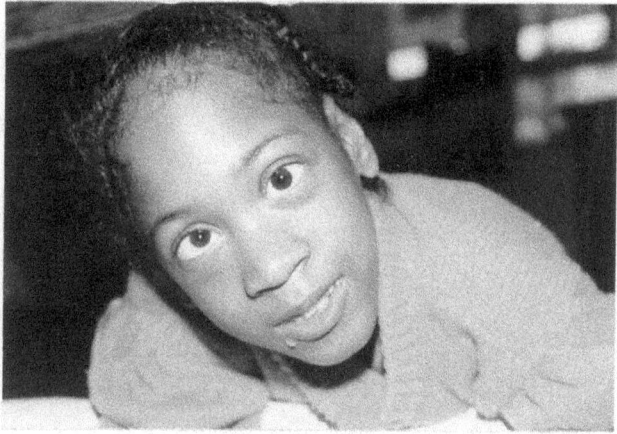

CHRISTINA

V. R. S. 2. C.

1988

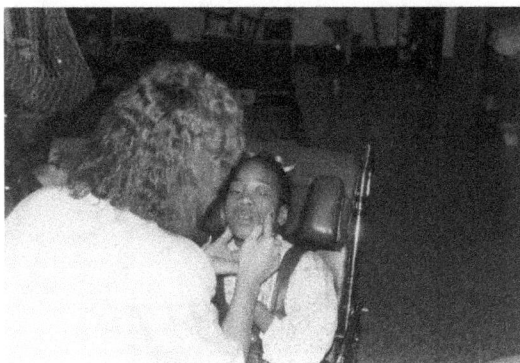

I am receiving oral-motor stimulation. This helps me swallow better.

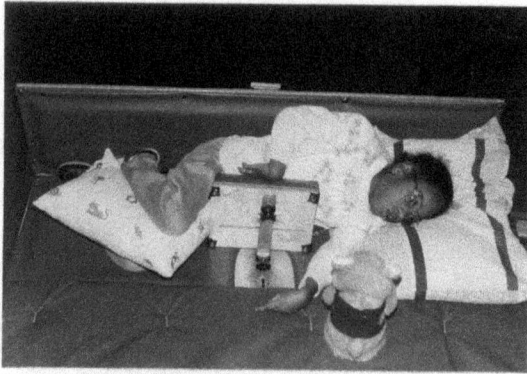

The sidelyer keeps my body in a good position. Gravity, pillows and the sidelyer all work together to straighten my back and get my body in the proper alignment.

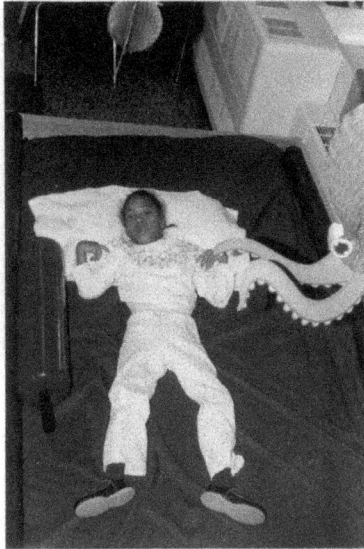

One of my favorite places to be is the water bed.

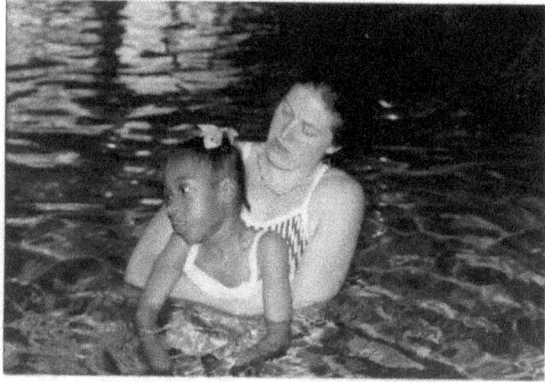

Another fun activity is the
swimming pool. It's fun to stand
up in the pool. I also work on
splashing with my hands and I really
kick my feet too!

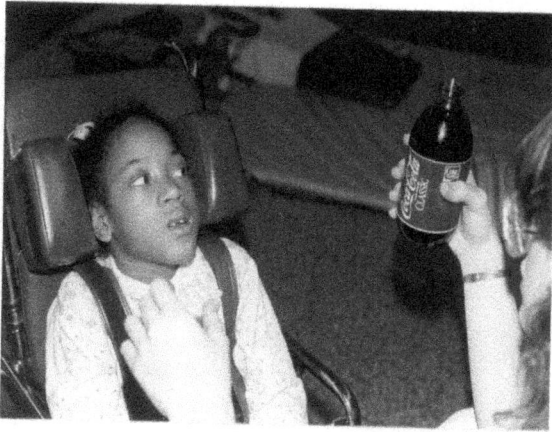

I have to make a choice between the cracker and the Coke. I really want the Coke so I look at it to let Scottie know that's what I want.

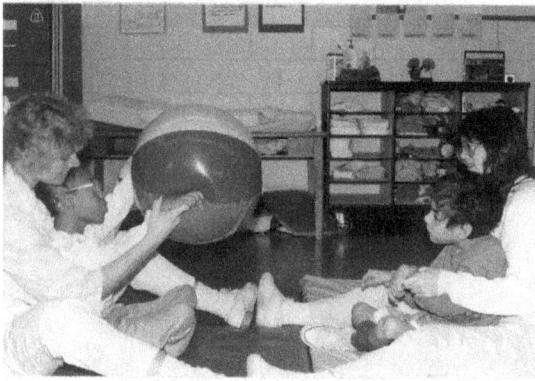

I am playing a game of
catch in P.E. with my friend Skye.

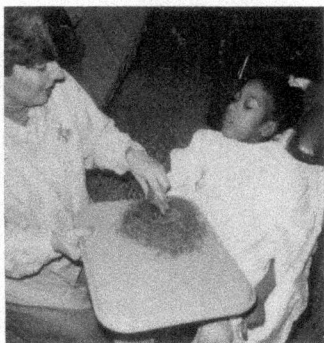

Making shamrocks for St.
Patrick's Day in Art class.

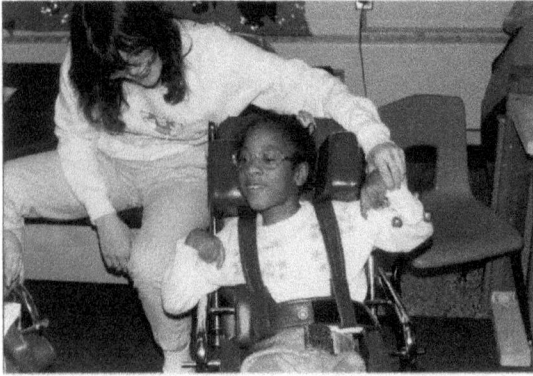

I am shaking the bells
in music and having such a good
time.

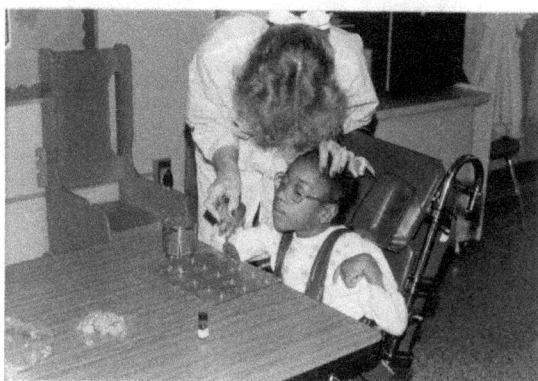

Making candy for our
Easter baskets was fun. I enjoyed
eating it even more!

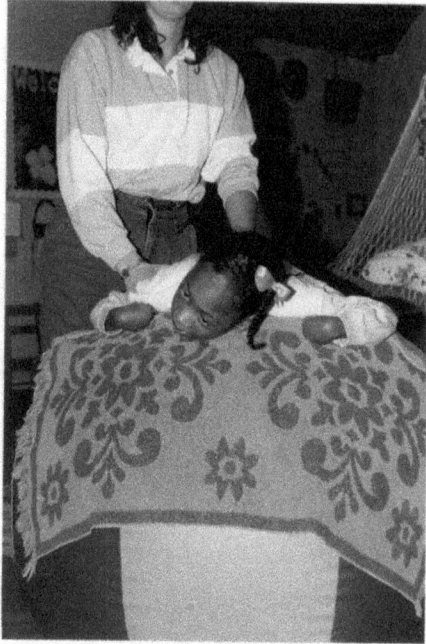

I am working over the therapy ball. I work hard on head control.

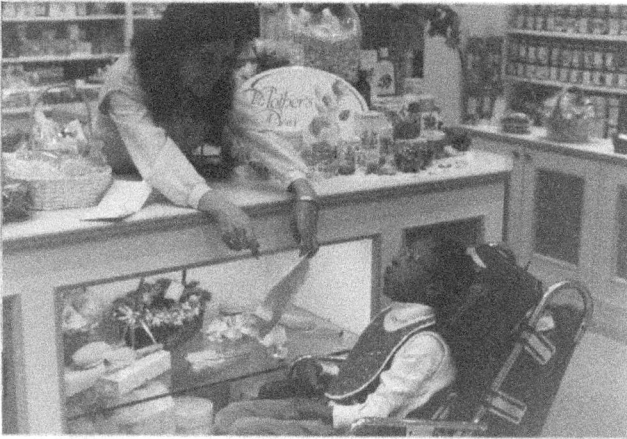

I hope Mom likes the gift
I bought her for Mother's Day. I
got it when we were out on
community integration. Surprise!

Happy Mother's Day!

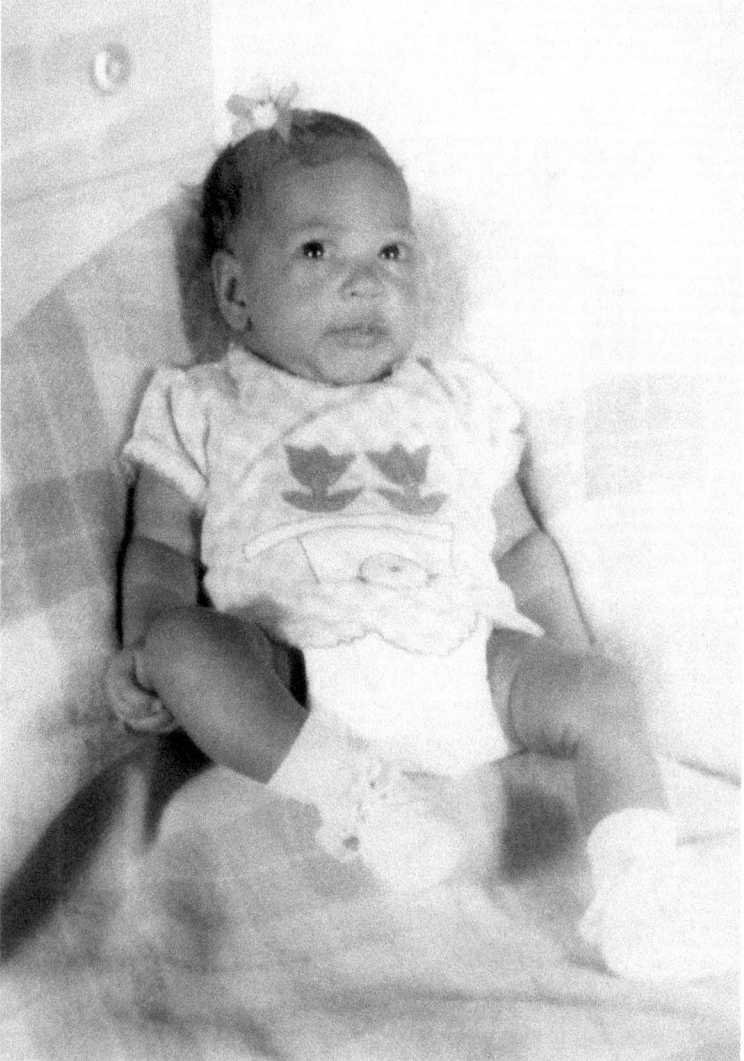

Christina, my sweet baby at 7 weeks old

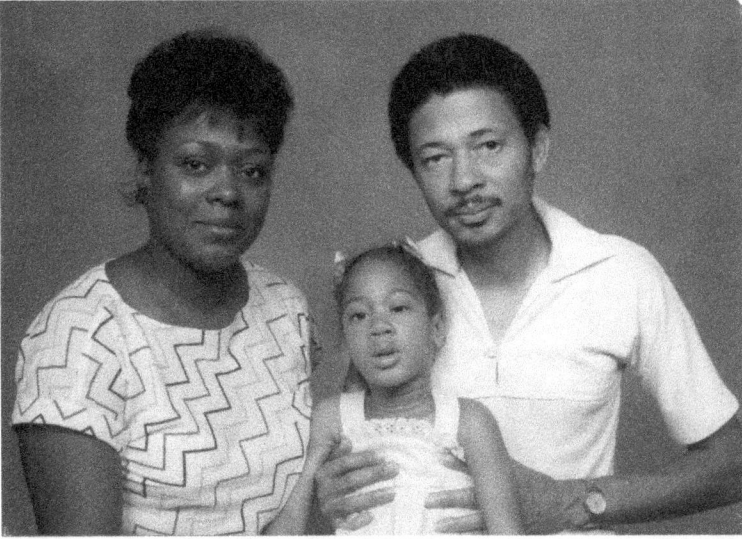

Stephanie, William and Christina Fortune, Our Lady of Lords Church, 1980

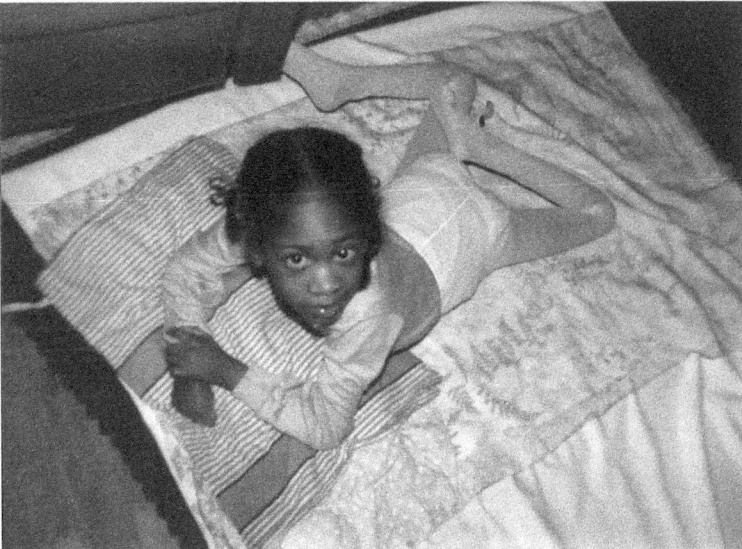

Relaxing on the floor, after her in-home therapy session, 7 years old.

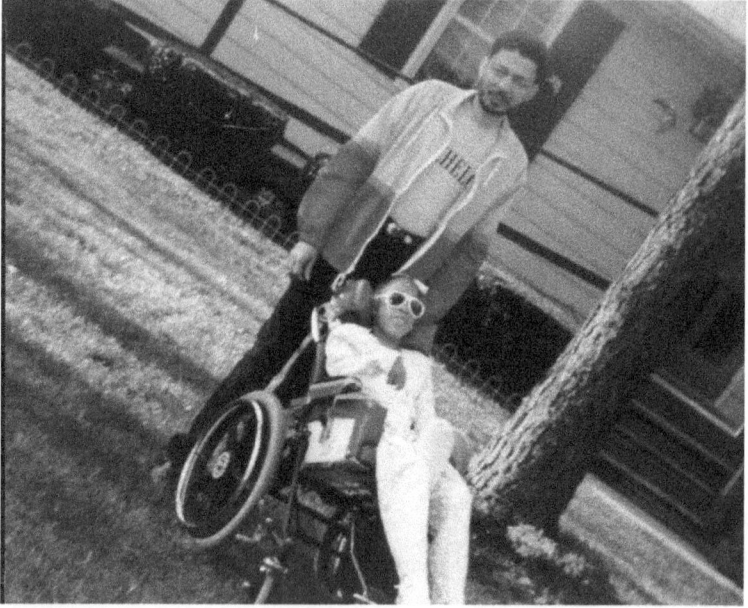

The must-have lime green outfit with her Dad, Easter Sunday 1987

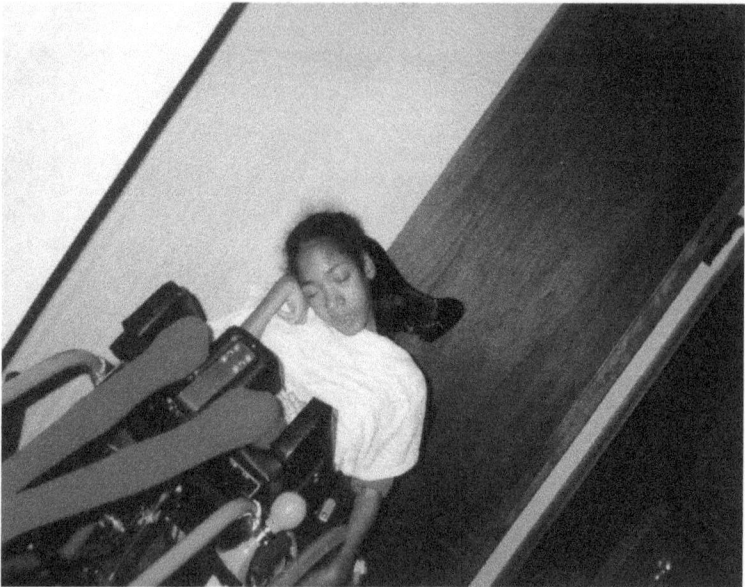

Nap time

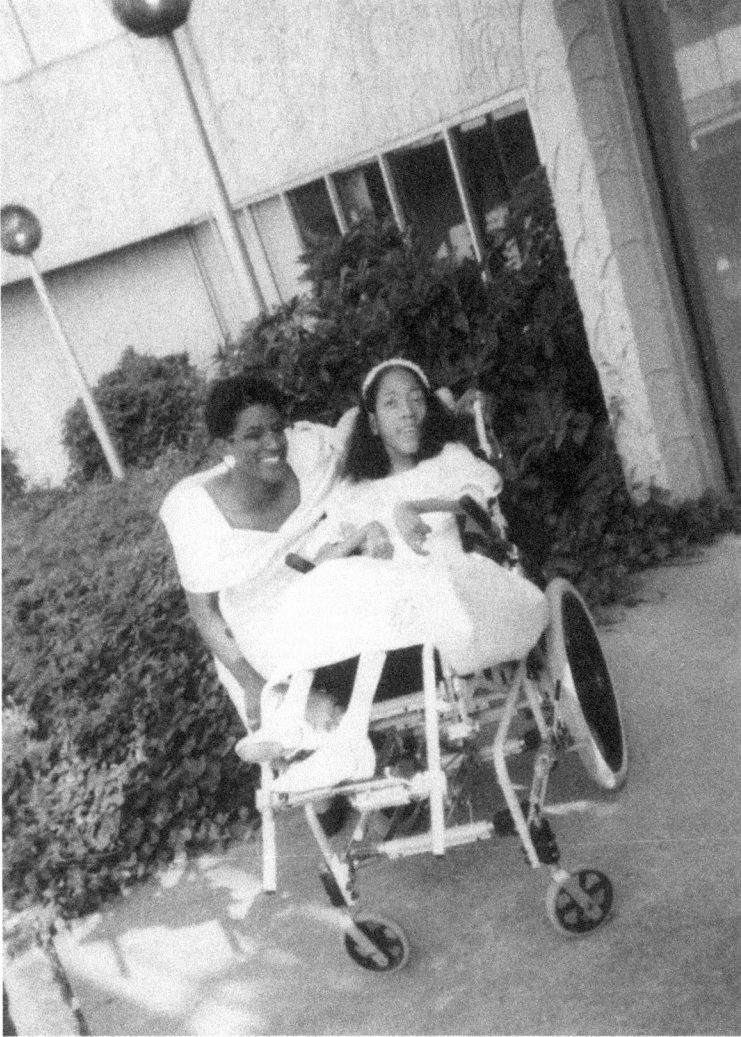

Christina and Rosa (family friend) at a wedding.

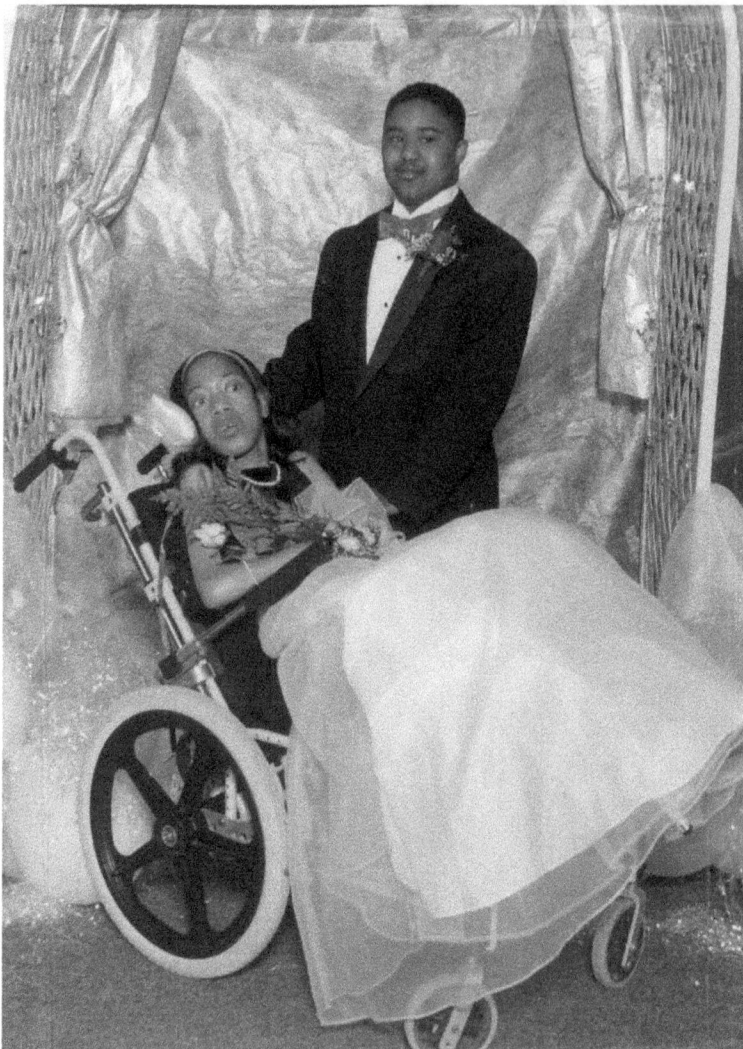

Christina and David on prom night, King William High School, 1999

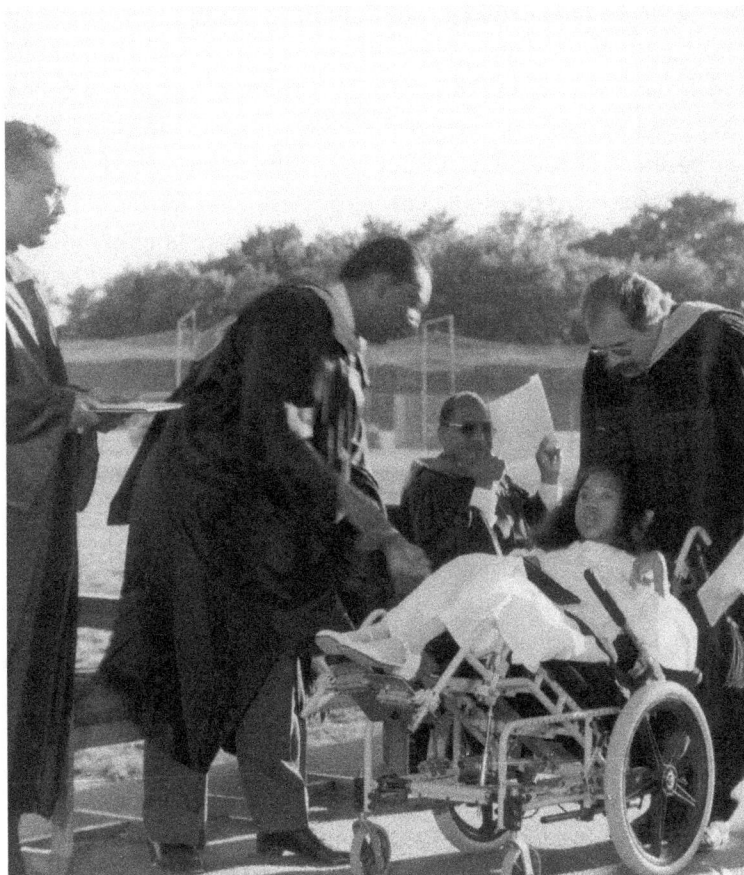

Getting her diploma on graduation day, surrounded by her teachers; Mr. Shipman stands behind her wheelchair.

in the summer. For her feet, I put white socks and Ked sneakers on her. Dark colors may make one sweat, and the dyes from the clothing can cause allergies. Cut out all tags or labels from the back of the clothing, as these can be irritating when left on.

Her hats were made from knit or cotton, and for winter, she had knit or fleece hats. Her caps did not have that hard plastic snap in the back of the cap because the snaps would pull her hair out and would be irritating to her head. I shopped for what I called "feel good fabrics" for feel-good clothing. This is what I looked for, because, of course, you want your child to look and feel good and be as clean as possible, just as you wish for yourself.

From time-to-time, drool would run from Christina's mouth, so I always made sure there were several small clean hand towels in her backpack. When she would drool, I would place a hand towel over her chest, and when she got on the school bus in the morning, I would fasten a hand towel to her coat. Her teacher helped do this by providing extra hand towels for school and in the van. Christina also had fancy towels for Christmas, Easter, her birthday and Valentine's Day.

Headrest: I made a cover made out of satin or silk for Christina's headrest on her wheelchair. This kept her hair on the back of her head smooth and kept her hair from being rubbed off the back and sides of her head.

The straps that came over her shoulders were covered with washable lambs' wool strap covers (available at Wal-mart in the car care section). The lambs' wool kept her straps from irritating her shoulder and the sides of her neck. When Christina's head was leaning along the side, her face lay on the softness of the lambs' wool.

Her armrest started to leave pressure marks on her arms so I bought gel bike seat covers (available in the bike section of Wal-mart). I also bought black shoestrings and made holes along the sides of the material edge of the gel seat covers. Be sure you are careful not to puncture holes in the gel. Put the shoestrings through the holes then fit the gel seat cover over each armrest until it is tight, keeping the shoestring and the knot away from

Christina's arm. The gel covers made a very nice soft topping for her arms to rest on. These gel seat covers can be used for lots of things for people in wheelchairs. They help prevent pressure marks. I would also place them on her foot rest when I removed her shoes.

Applesauce for Christina
Some of her favorite Dishes

Manna from Heaven – The Other Side to Angel Dust

Christina was truly a lover of good food. She loved to eat her vegetables, greens, chicken, chicken liver, and fish. Everything had to have a sauce made of tomatoes, cheese, brown gravy or a barbecue sauce.

Her favorite drinks were fruit drinks and most especially was the homemade smoothies. She liked her food soft, chopped or mashed because it was easier for her to eat. I used a mini plus food processor to mix her food. I never used plastic utensils because she could have bitten into the plastic and choked or swallowed the plastic. I would only give her flexible straws for her drinks, which avoided spills. Christina took seizure medications three times a day, and I used jams or jellies to mix together to give her the medication; the little jelly packs worked well (available from any restaurant that serves breakfast). What we had for dinner the night before, she also took for her school lunch.

Here are a few quick recipes that were Christina's favorites. You may like them for yourself.

(Note: When using condensed soups, always dilute with water or milk. You can use less water.)

Recipes

Fruit

Oh yes—fruit desserts. She loved hot spoon bread with homemade applesauce.

Homemade Applesauce
Peel apples
Take out the seeds and the core of the apple
Wash the pieces and put them into a pan.
Cover them halfway with apple juice.
Add a little butter
Sugar to taste
Pinch of cinnamon and nutmeg
1 cap full of vanilla extract
Cook until tender or soft
Mash or chop for chunky applesauce
You can make it with peach, apricot, or pear—whatever you have a taste for when making this dish. Christina had a hard time passing her bowels so eating this would help. After school or before bedtime, I gave her a warm bowl of fruit sauce. She also liked plum sauce made from prunes. If you do not want to use sugar, you can use honey. Sometimes I put her sauces over oatmeal or Cream of Wheat for added flavor. I also mixed them in milk or yogurt drinks. You can also mash a banana or strawberries or other fruit to taste. If you like it thick use less water or juice.

Apple and Sweet Potatoes
In a saucepan, add 1 cup of water, butter, sugar or honey, pinch of cinnamon and nutmeg, ½ cap-full each of vanilla and lemon extract. Cut up 1 sweet potato and 1 apple. Cover and cook until tender, about 20 to 25 minutes.

Smoothie Fruit Drink
1 cup of yogurt
½ cup of milk
1/3 cup of orange juice
Add mashed banana and strawberries. To make it thicker, add ice cream. Blend altogether. Enjoy!

Spoon Bread with Apples (or fruit of your choice)
1 box of spoon bread mix (Martha Washington is what I use)
Follow recipe on box. Just add in chopped apples. Bake and serve warm with lots of butter.

Jell-O and Puréed Fruit
1 pack of flavored Jell-O
1 cup hot water
1 cup cold water
Add ½ cup of puree fruit sauce
Chill for several hours

Cream of Wheat and Eggs (topped with applesauce)
Cook cream of wheat and put into a bowl. Scramble an egg and add cheese. Place over cream of wheat and top with applesauce. Serve warm.

Cream of Wheat Shake (You can also use oatmeal)
Cook cream of wheat and add butter, sugar (or honey) to taste while cream of wheat is cooking. After cooking, put cereal into a ½ glass of milk. Add pureed fruit or a mashed banana or strawberries. You can use a straw with this. Stir and enjoy warm or cool.

Vegetables and Meat

Honey Glazed Carrots
2 lbs. carrots (scraped and thinly sliced)
½ cup water
3 tablespoons honey
3 tablespoons brown sugar
2 tablespoons butter
Combine carrots and water in a saucepan. Bring to a boil, then cover and simmer for approximately 10 minutes or until tender. Drain off water and add honey and other ingredients. Cover, low heat, stirring until butter and sugar melts.

Cheesy Broccoli and Stuffed Potatoes (you can stuff potatoes with chicken or fish also)
1 large baking potato
Bake potato in oven or microwave. Cut open, mash inside of potato, and add butter, salt and a little pepper. Chop chicken or fish and add to mashed inside of potato. Cover with cooked broccoli and top with a cheesy sauce.

Cheesy Potato Casserole (you can add chicken or ham)
7 medium-diced potatoes
¼ cup butter (melted)
1 small chopped onion
Pinch of salt and pepper
1 carton of sour cream
1 can cream of chicken soup (undiluted)
2 cups shredded cheddar cheese
Extra 3 tablespoons butter (melted)
1 ½-cup herb of seasoned stuffing mix
Dice potatoes and cook in boiling water until tender; drain and let cool. Combine ¼ cup of butter and next 5 ingredients in a large bowl. Gently stir in potatoes and cheese. Spoon into a lightly greased 13 x 9 x 2-inch baking dish. Combine 3 tablespoons butter and stuffing mix. Sprinkle over potato mixture. Bake uncovered

at 350 degrees for 25 minutes or until thoroughly heated. It is wonderful. When I cooked this, I had to send extra to Christina's school.

Cabbage, Corned Beef and Potatoes

1 large cabbage (chopped)
1 small onion
Salt and pepper to taste
Butter
3 large potatoes, diced
1 can corn beef

In a large saucepan with top, add 2 cups of water. Add potatoes, salt, pepper and chop onion and butter. Cook for approximately 15 minutes until potatoes are tender. Add chopped cabbage and corned beef and cook covered for 15 minutes more. You may have to cook the cabbage a little longer for someone with special needs like Christina. Her cabbage had to be soft in order for her to eat it. I had to use the food processor to chop the cabbage.

Old Fashioned Macaroni and Cheese

1 package elbow macaroni
2 ½ cups shredded cheddar cheese
1 ½ cups milk
2 large eggs, lightly beaten
1 teaspoon salt
1/8 teaspoon pepper

Cook macaroni according to package directions; drain. Make a layer 1/3 of macaroni in a lightly greased 2 quart casserole dish; sprinkle with 1/3 cheese, then repeat and top with remaining macaroni (reserve remaining cheese).

Combine milk, eggs, salt and pepper. Pour over macaroni and cheese. Cover and bake at 350 degrees for 45 minutes. Uncover and sprinkle with remaining cheese and paprika. Cover and let stand 10 minutes before serving.

Stove-top Chicken Bake

1 package stove top stuffing mix for chicken
1 ½ lb. boneless, skinless chicken breast, cut into 1-inch pieces
1 can condensed cream of chicken soup
1/3 cup sour cream
1 bag 16 oz. frozen mixed vegetables, thawed and drained

Preheat oven to 400 degrees. Prepare stuffing mix as directed on package and set aside. Mix chicken soup, sour cream and vegetables in a 13 x9 inch baking dish. Top with the stuffing. Bake 30 minutes or until chicken is cooked through. Really good!

Turnip and Bacon

4 or 5 large turnips
1 small onion
Pinch of sugar
Salt and pepper
5 slices of fried bacon and grease

Cut up turnip and place in a saucepan and cover with water, add chopped onion, sugar salt and pepper. After cooking bacon, add all of it to the cooking turnips after chopping up bacon. Cover and cook for 30 minutes or until the water has cooked down and the turnips are tender. Very tasty!

Carrot Pudding

2 cups mashed cooked carrots
1 cup milk
½ cup sugar
Pinch of salt
3 tablespoons butter
Pinch of nutmeg
2 eggs

Add milk, sugar, salt, butter, nutmeg and carrots together. Beat until fluffy. Beat eggs into mixture then pour into greased baking dish. Bake at 350 degrees for 50 to 60 minutes or until firm. Top with a dusting of confectioner's sugar.

Asparagus with Cheese Sauce

Cook asparagus in butter and cover with cheese sauce. Christina liked this with fish.

Gourmet Mashed Potatoes and Chicken Livers

4 large potatoes
1 can cream of chicken soup
1 package chicken livers, stir fried
1 stick of butter
½ cup milk
Salt and pepper to taste
Stir fried chicken livers and one small onion in butter. 1 box broccoli, chopped, cooked and drained. Cook potatoes, mash them, then add all ingredients. Put into a large bowl and top with chicken livers, onions and broccoli.

Spinach Quiche

1 – 10 oz. package frozen chopped spinach
½ pint sour cream
4 oz. can mushroom pieces (optional)
4 oz. grated cheddar cheese
3 large eggs
Sauté mushrooms in butter. Cook and drain spinach. Mix sour cream and eggs. Fold everything together in a bowl. Pour into greased 9-inch pie plate. Bake at 350 degrees until eggs are set for about 30-45 minutes.

Creamed Spinach

1 package frozen chopped spinach, thawed and drained
½ cup sour cream
½ cup parmesan cheese
2 cans cream of potato soup
½ cup shredded Monterey Jack cheese
Mix all ingredients, except jack cheese, in a bowl. Pour into baking dish; sprinkle on top with jack cheese. Bake at 350 degrees for 30-35 minutes or until cheese bubbles.

Scalloped Tuna and Potatoes

5 cooked potatoes
1 - 7 oz. can tuna
1 tablespoon diced onion
1 can condensed celery soup
Paprika

Slice potatoes and flake tuna. Grease casserole dish and fill with alternate layers of potatoes, tuna, and onion and celery soup until all are used. Pour the oil from tuna over mixture and sprinkle with paprika. Bake in hot oven at 425 degrees for approximately 30 minutes.

Aunt Nellie's Harvard Beets (sweet & sour).

You can buy it already in the jar.

I hope you enjoy these recipes. These were a few of Christina's favorite dishes. Your whole family will enjoy them just as mine did.

God Bless You!

Stephanie Fortune

www.ingramcontent.com/pod-product-compliance
Lightning Source LLC
Chambersburg PA
CBHW021916190326
41519CB00008B/795